Surviving Lung Cancer

(My Story)

By

Darlene Lehosit

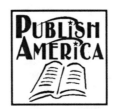

PublishAmerica
Baltimore

First printing

ISBN: 1-4241-6344-7
PUBLISHED BY PUBLISHAMERICA, LLLP
www.publishamerica.com
Baltimore

Printed in the United States of America

DEDICATION

To all cancer survivors and cancer patients everywhere; to Dr. Edward Harris, my oncologist at the Fountain Valley Cancer Center in Fountain Valley, California; Dr. James Roberts, my oncologist at the Mary Babb Randolph Cancer Center at West Virginia University in Morgantown, West Virginia; to Jane Urso, who heads up my cancer support group and who has been a great inspiration to me; and last, but not least, to Joe, my husband, my soul mate, without whose encouragement I might never have finished this book.

ACKNOWLEDGEMENTS

I would like to acknowledge Bryan School of Court Reporting in Los Angeles without which I would not have had the tenacity, persistence, fortitude, and endurance to complete this book.

To Anna Egan Smucker without whose recommendation I would not have been led to PublishAmerica.

To my publisher, PublishAmerica, for undertaking this project.

To all cancer patients everywhere. There is hope.

To my husband Joe without whom I would not have survived my ordeal. I love you.

INTRODUCTION

I first met Darlene Lehosit in August of 2001 when she moved from California to West Virginia and I began to follow her for small cell carcinoma of the lung. Her cancer presented with a history of chronic cough. X-rays showed a left hilar mass which spread to the lymph nodes in the center of the chest and right lobe of the liver. Mrs. Lehosit was treated in California with six cycles of chemotherapy and has remained in complete remission from her cancer at the present time. It is highly unusual for patients with small cell lung cancer that has spread to the liver to live five years and be cured of their cancer. Mrs. Lehosit is an energetic woman with a positive outlook on life. It seems to me that her outcome is due to the excellent care she received with her oncologist in California and her strong faith.

John S. Rogers II, M.D.
Professor of Medicine
Medical Co-Director
Sara Crile Allen & John Frederick Allen
Comprehensive Lung Cancer Program
Mary Babb Randolph Cancer Center
Morgantown, West Virginia

PREFACE

Cancer patients share a bond, born of necessity. To travel in the unknown land of cancer survivorship, one needs wise companions, and it is through other cancer patients that they seem to find the wisdom and support they so desperately need.

When Darlene Lehosit first came to our cancer support group, I had no idea how profoundly she would influence the lives of everyone in the room. Quiet, unassuming, she took her place among us and over the next months began to share her story. As that story unfolded, all of us realized we were in the presence of a miracle.

A diagnosis which involves only a 10% probability of surviving is little less than a death sentence. With such a disease, treatment is as debilitating as the disease itself. The struggle to survive is, at best, an uphill battle. Darlene has been able to survive not only cancer, but also the repeated painful bouts with gout. In her suffering, she has triumphed. She is cancer-free and she has chosen to freely share the wisdom she has gained.

Her decision to write her story was a courageous one. To be willing to dig deeply into oneself and explore for the benefit of others is a mark of true wisdom. Darlene's story is one of hope. In spite of the long odds, she has not only survived, but blossomed. Her joy in living, her giving of herself through her volunteer work and her testimony to her deep faith serve as beacons to those whose journey will take them into the depths of battling cancer.

I am deeply grateful to her for sharing her story and providing hope for those of us who know her. Now it is time for her story to touch those beyond our small group. I joyfully applaud her effort and am certain the story of our miracle lady will inspire all who read these pages.

Jane W. Urso

CHAPTER ONE

This book will have accomplished what I set out for it to do if just one person gains some strength and the ability to fight to get through his or her treatment for cancer, be it chemotherapy, radiation, or whatever modality of treatment it is that person is undergoing.

My name is Darlene Lehosit, and I was diagnosed with small-cell metastatic carcinoma on February 19, 1999.

For many years I'd had a prior history of upper respiratory problems and had been diagnosed with allergic asthma. My journey into the world of cancer began with some very simple and very common symptoms which could have easily been mistaken for asthma-related problems.

After cleaning the bathroom one morning with a powerful cleanser, I developed a cough. I did not, however, relate this cough to using the strong cleanser. The cough grew worse as the days passed. Fatigue was prevalent, also, during this time. I found that I became extremely tired in the afternoons. When I was home working on my computer during the day, it was a common occurrence for me to lean back in my comfortable high-back leather chair, close my eyes, and fall sound asleep. Other times I would get up and go lie down on our bed, and I would sleep for one or two hours. It should be noted that I was never one to take a nap in the afternoons, no matter how tired I was.

Very soon I began to cough and could not stop coughing, no matter how many cough drops I had nor how much water I would drink when the coughing began. I decided, since it was wintertime and it did not appear to be my yearly cold coming on, that I would call Dr. Weissman, my allergist, and go see him. I was told upon calling Dr. Weissman's office that he was out of town at a medical conference, so I called Dr. Johnson instead, who was my general practitioner. He had originally referred me to Dr. Weissman; so since the two of them were in consultation with one another regarding their mutual patients, Dr. Johnson was very familiar with my medical history relating to the asthma and also the treatment I was undergoing with Dr. Weissman.

It was urgent that I see Dr. Johnson right away because my husband and I had planned a trip to Laughlin, Nevada, along with two lady friends. We had intended to drive our motor homes and set up camp in an RV park across the river from the casinos. Dr. Johnson prescribed some medication for my coughing which had worked for me in the past. He told me if the desert winds kicked up once we arrived, as they are prone to do, for me to take the medicine, that it should relieve any problem I might have with coughing. So when it came time to go, we left home in anticipation of having a great weekend.

The RV park was in Bullhead City, Arizona. We had a terrific view of all the lights twinkling at night, inviting everyone to come into the casinos and take a chance on their game of choice. It was a beautiful RV park which we enjoyed, and all of us looked forward to doing some sightseeing while we were there.

We had a wonderful time the first evening with our friends, and I was able to join everybody for a drink and some people-watching in one of the casino lounges. The next day we had planned to see the town of Laughlin, Nevada, and some of the other nearby towns. I was understandably concerned because by this time my cough had become very persistent and was causing me a tremendous amount of discomfort and overwhelming fatigue. I would double over when I began coughing, while at the same time holding my sides because they ached unbearably every time I tried to breathe, let alone cough.

It didn't take much soul-searching on my part to realize that I was not able to join everyone when they ventured out to see the sights. To make matters worse, the wind had kicked up, and as many of you may know from firsthand experience, the wind created a good deal of dust in the air. I stayed in the motor home and slept between attacks of coughing, and I was once again overcome with fatigue. I thought the cough would go away after taking the medication that Dr. Johnson had prescribed for me, but it did not; it only seemed to exacerbate the problem.

We came home the next morning, and as soon as I was able, I made an appointment to see Dr. Johnson because of my concern that my problem was much more serious than a common cold or an allergic reaction to something.

CHAPTER TWO

Dr. Johnson scheduled chest X-rays initially. He sent me to Dr. Klein, a radiologist whom I had been seeing for yearly mammograms since arriving in Southern California. In fact, I had been seeing both of these doctors for a period of over twenty years. Dr. Klein's medical report indicated that there appeared to be a shadow behind my heart.

Dr. Johnson prescribed getting an MRI done in order to discover what the shadow was behind my heart and also to begin an in-depth search of what was causing my problem. However, prior to the MRI, Dr. Johnson had recommended a bronchoscopy to see if, in fact, they could see a tumor in the lung; and after several discussions with Dr. Sommers, the doctor performing the bronchoscopy, he said that they could not detect any growth within the bronchi, and he felt that if, in fact, it was a tumor, it was not protruding into the bronchi, in lay terms, the sacs in the lungs.

It was after the bronchoscopy test that Dr. Johnson felt there still should be some additional testing performed because, although he didn't say it to me, I believe at this time that he thought the shadow behind my heart was, indeed, a tumor in the chest cavity, which the MRI did, in fact, reveal.

Dr. Johnson requested that a sonogram be performed to see if possibly the tumor could have metastasized to another soft-tissue organ, such as the liver. The result of the sonogram showed that there was some irregularity in my liver which the medical personnel doing the sonogram referred to as a spot.

The next test I underwent was the final test, the brutal, virtually inhumane (I know of no other way to describe it) test called a liver biopsy.

CHAPTER THREE

The tests I had undergone up to this point, the chest X-ray, the bronchoscopy, the MRI, had not been that invasive nor particularly painful except maybe for the bronchoscopy, which allows a physician to examine inside your airway for any abnormality such as foreign bodies, bleeding, et cetera. Although that test was extremely uncomfortable, there is still no way I could nor would ever compare it to the liver biopsy.

During the bronchoscopy a tube or tubes (I can't remember which) was/were inserted into my bronchial cavity, which, as I said, is very uncomfortable. By doing this examination the doctor was able to see if there were any obstructions in the bronchial cavity. None were observed.

As the doctors proceeded with all of these tests, I, of course, became very apprehensive of the possibility that I may have cancer. All medical personnel were careful not to mention the word "cancer," but surely that possibility must have been in the back of their minds, also.

I'd never had reason to have a liver biopsy performed before, and I was not prepared for all the pain I was to endure during the procedure. I was admitted to the hospital as an outpatient, as I was told that I would only be there for a few hours. When they wheeled me into the test room, I was instructed to lie on the table which was part of a CT scan machine.

The doctor, whose name I do not recall, introduced himself to me and proceeded to explain a little bit about the test. The first thing I asked him is if he was going to put me to sleep. You can imagine that I was very uneasy at this point. It seems he expected me to follow the instructions he gave me while I was awake: "Breathe"; "Hold your breath"; "Let it out." He said I had to lie perfectly still while he injected a needle, which appeared to me to be two feet long at the time, into my abdominal area. With this needle the doctor performing the liver biopsy would puncture my liver by way of the abdominal wall and be able to retrieve a sample or samples to be biopsied by the doctor who entered the procedure room a little bit later and whom I assumed to be the pathologist. At the same time the doctor performing the liver biopsy would be doing this I would undergo a CT scan, which would be taking pictures of my liver. This procedure is more commonly referred to as a CAT scan. In medical jargon that is Computerized Axial Tomography. Most of us laymen know this procedure as a CT scan.

Because of the coughing jags that would come and go randomly, before the procedure began I asked the nurse if the doctor intended to give me a sedative of some kind, and she said no, that he did not. So I immediately told her that the coughing had a tendency to start at any time, and when it did, I had no control over it, and I mentioned how it would double me over, and how could I possibly lie perfectly still and cooperate with the test when that was happening?! I literally begged her to ask him to give me something to calm my nerves. She told the doctor what I had related to her and asked him if he would give me a sedative. Thankfully he agreed to do so.

In spite of being administered the sedative, my entire body was trembling so hard from stress at this time that I couldn't imagine all of this occurring the way the doctor expected it to. I have no memory of it, but surely he must have injected a topical pain medication into my abdominal area before proceeding with the liver biopsy.

He penetrated the abdominal cavity with the two-foot long needle and proceeded to take more than one sample from my liver. Then before I knew it he disappeared and returned shortly thereafter with another doctor who had to have been the pathologist. The doctor performing the procedure took more liver samples, and the two doctors huddled together over a small table where these samples were deposited, quietly discussing what they were seeing. I could not hear them, so I asked the doctor performing my procedure what they saw. He told me to contact my own physician, that Dr. Johnson would have the results of the test in a day or so.

The liver biopsy was a very painful experience. Every time the doctor repeated penetration of my abdominal cavity and went back in there with that needle, I literally had to do everything in my power to stop myself from screaming. The table was soaking wet with my perspiration when the test was over, which is probably no surprise to anyone reading this. I was never so glad to get a test over with as I was this liver biopsy.

My allergist, Dr. Weissman, was heavily involved in research at UC Irvine in Orange County where we lived. Of course, he knew that I'd undergone a liver biopsy. During one of our visits he told me that he and some other doctors were involved in research which was going to involve a liver biopsy. Because he was aware that I'd undergone this particular procedure, he asked me what I thought would be a fair amount of money to offer somebody to volunteer to undergo a liver biopsy for the medical study that he was about to become involved in. He wanted to know if $500 would be a sufficient amount of money to offer a volunteer to undergo this test. In other words, knowing what I know now, would I volunteer to undergo a liver biopsy for that amount of money. I told him absolutely not. Then he proceeded to ask me if I thought $1,000 would be a sufficient amount of money to offer somebody to undergo this procedure, and I said no. In fact, I told Dr. Weissman, having undergone a liver biopsy and knowing what transpires during this procedure, that I would not volunteer for $5,000, not even for $10,000, because, in my opinion, it was simply too painful, not to mention too stressful an experience.

Although the liver biopsy was physically unpleasant, dreadfully painful and one of the most horrific experiences I've ever had to undergo in my entire lifetime (I'm now 63 years old), I can look back and realize that the results of this procedure were positive and detected the cancer, which led to the diagnosis of the disease, which led to my receiving the proper care and treatment, which led to its ultimately going into remission.

During my next visit with Dr. Johnson, my general practitioner, he told me the liver biopsy had revealed that I had small-cell metastatic carcinoma of the lung and that it had metastasized to the liver. When he relayed the diagnosis to me, I felt as though I'd had been dealt a severe blow to the solar plexus. The wind seemed to have been knocked right out of me. Life itself seemed to stand still, and I found myself without a voice. I literally could not speak. Upon my being told that I had been diagnosed with cancer, Dr. Johnson said that he had made an appointment for me with an oncologist, Dr. Edward Harris.

Immediately after hearing the diagnosis, my eyes filled with tears, but I do not remember crying in Dr. Johnson's office. I nodded in the affirmative when he asked me if I was okay, which was far from true, and when he asked if I wanted him to call somebody to come and be with me, I just shook my head no. When I was at the front desk checking out, the receptionist asked me if I was okay, and because I still could not find my voice, I shook my head no, and I felt the tears filling my eyes; then I left. Before I reached my car the tears came pouring out, and they wouldn't stop for a very long while. I called my husband Joe as soon as I returned to the car to let him know the results of the tests. Of course, he offered all the love and support that he could over the telephone, and tried to reassure me that it would be all right, we would do what had to be done and that we would get through this together.

CHAPTER FOUR

The day after the liver biopsy came back positive, my husband and I sat outside of the Fountain Valley Cancer Center in Fountain Valley, California, for what seemed like a very long time before going inside where we would have our initial meeting with Dr. Harris, the man who was to become my oncologist. Before going into the medical building Joe put his arms around me and reassured me that together we would do whatever it takes to beat this disease. Through my tears I couldn't have agreed more. At that moment I wanted very much to be well again.

Overcoming cancer is a very individual experience, but you are blessed indeed if you have a spouse as loving and wonderful as mine, or a relative or dear friend who will be part of your support group while you undergo treatment because treatment, for me at least, was more traumatic than anything I've ever experienced in my entire lifetime. With the exception of the liver biopsy, of course. I really don't see how anything will ever surpass that experience.

I have always had a very strong faith in God, and I can tell you honestly that I did not once ask Him that inevitable question: "Why me?" Rather, I asked Him for the strength I would need to do His will, and to get through the coming months. What I did was put myself in God's hands because I knew that I had absolutely no control over what was to happen next. I also found myself asking Him to take me into His arms and to offer me comfort because oftentimes I would find myself at the depths of despair, and I believed that only He could provide the comfort that I was seeking, that I desperately needed. I am confident that my having cancer brought me closer to Him than I'd ever been before, so much so that I found myself having conversations with Him on a personal level much the same as I am talking to you now. Speaking to Him became a daily ritual with me, and remains so to this day. I would also pray the rosary each day because it gave me a remarkable peace of mind, and I believe I gained an enormous amount of inner strength by doing so.

Today my conversations with Him consist mainly of my thanking Him for another beautiful day, for giving my life back to me, and for the many blessings that have been bestowed on me. Even if a Nor'easter is blowing a gale outside and it's snowing to beat the band, to every cancer survivor it's a beautiful day. For the benefit of the people not living on the East Coast, a Nor'easter is a very severe storm originating in Canada which has crossed our border and is literally raising havoc outdoors.

It is said that having the proper mental attitude is a great asset in helping a person overcome cancer or some other debilitating disease, for that matter. And I agree with that theory one hundred per cent. I most definitely had the will to live. I went in the oncologist's office on that morning of February 19, 1999, with the attitude that I was going to come out of treatment cancer-free. Although difficult at times, this is the attitude I carried with me throughout the six months of my chemotherapy. Yes, I was put to the test often during treatment, and I sunk to depths of depression so low that I didn't think I could possibly sink any lower. But with all my might I tried not to waver; I tried rather to concentrate on how good life was going to be once I became well again.

Before our first meeting with Dr. Harris began, my husband and I met and spoke with a counselor employed by his office. The purpose of this meeting, which lasted approximately 45 minutes, was to do the mundane things that you do when you meet with a doctor for the first time, such as fill out the insurance forms. At this time the counselor gathered all of my biographical information. She also counseled me a little bit on the subject of cancer, the treatment, how many people survive chemotherapy, and she told me that there are many different types of cancer. She said that the rate of survival is good, and not to believe all the horror stories we hear about cancer. It was a very informative meeting, intended to be of some comfort to me. However, I cannot say that I felt comforted because I was still reeling from the shock I'd experienced in Dr. Johnson's office the previous day when he informed me that I had cancer.

My first meeting with Dr. Harris was very nerve-racking, to say the least, mostly because of my fear of cancer, fear of the unknown, and what lies ahead.

First appearances can be deceiving, as they were in this case. Dr. Harris didn't look a day over 25, and yet he was a professor of oncology at the University of Southern California at Los Angeles, and very renown and respected in his field of medicine. Dr. Johnson had highly recommended him. I was very grateful that he had because, as I learned once I began my treatment under his care, Dr. Harris would prove in the months to come to be a very consoling and comforting figure, as well as being a take-charge, no-nonsense kind of doctor, the kind I was happy to have on my side during this very trying period in my life.

Dr. Harris had an extremely positive discussion with me and my husband, and he told us that in cases similar to mine, the recovery rate for a patient with a tumor such as the one he saw behind my heart was ninety per cent. This, of course, being contrary to our discussion six months later, after my treatments had ceased when Dr. Harris informed me that only ten per cent of the patients with the kind of cancer I had survive. Thank goodness he chose the tack that he did. Dr. Harris was relaying this information in order to give hope to both of us, and it worked very well in my case because I thought often about what he said, thinking I stood a very good chance of overcoming this dreadful disease, all I had to do was grin and bear the chemotherapy treatments as best I could. Realistically, I also knew there was always the possibility that I could lose the battle, and that is where I relied upon my faith in God, praying for the strength I would need to get through the coming months and the strength to do His will, whatever it may be.

Dr. Harris had been forwarded the results of all the tests, and I presented him with my latest chest X-rays during our consultation. The X-rays showed what might be described as a large shadow behind the heart. That shadow, as it turns out, was the tumor. When the liver biopsy came back positive, it indicated that the tumor had metastasized to the liver, meaning the cancer had traveled to the liver from the left lung, so it was well on its way to doing what small-cell metastatic carcinoma does, it travels to other soft-tissue organs of the body via the bloodstream.

It was less than thirty minutes into our meeting with Dr. Harris when he told my husband and me that without a doubt the cancer was caused from smoking. I had tried for many years to quit smoking, and finally succeeded with the help of a hypnotist fifteen years prior to that time, but obviously the damage had already been done.

CHAPTER FIVE

I had smoked cigarettes for many years, twenty-five years, to be exact. I tried to quit more times than I can count without very much success. At the time I started smoking the Surgeon General did not issue warnings on packs of cigarettes, and just about everybody I knew enjoyed smoking back then. Certainly none more than I. I was totally addicted to cigarettes, as I realized when I tried to quit those many times on my own without success. Even the promise by my wonderful husband of a brand-new car of my choice did not deter my smoking.

We bought the car, with my promise that I would stop smoking, and once again I attempted to give up the cigarettes. I was hopelessly addicted; and for a while, even after I started smoking again, I didn't do so in the new car. That did not last for very long, however, and before I realized it the ashtray was overflowing with cigarette ashes and butts. Why are smokers so frightfully untidy? It's no wonder smoking is referred to as a dirty habit. I'll go one step further and refer to it as a filthy habit.

My job as a freelance court reporter was a very high-stress job. I was in this profession for twenty-two years; and I had convinced myself that smoking eased some of the stress that went along with the job because during the breaks from taking down testimony on my Stenograph machine, I would enjoy smoking a cigarette. I finally was able to quit some years later after just one visit to a hypnotist.

Before entering the hypnotist's office the first thing I saw was a tiny baby's coffin (it looked very much like a regulation baby's coffin to me), and it was filled with sand and cigarette butts, lots of them. It was here that the patients of this hypnotist would snuff out what they hoped would be their last cigarette before their visit with this doctor. I guarantee you that the image of that infant's coffin filled with sand and cigarette butts is something I shall never forget. It left an imprint on my mind that will be with me as long as I live. The vision of those cigarette butts in the sand of that coffin is in my mind's eye today just as clearly as it was the day I first saw it.

What I recall about my visit with the hypnotist is his putting me under hypnosis, and proceeding by power of suggestion to have me take a journey down a very long flight of steps. I was instructed to begin descending the stairs very slowly and to continue until I reached the bottom. All of this time the hypnotist was talking to me, I suppose convincing me just how bad smoking was for me and instilling in my mind that I should and could quit this devastating habit if I really wanted to. I can't remember what occurred during this session other than what I have related here; but that is typical of being put under hypnosis, you are instructed at the end of the session to remember nothing that was said during the time you've spent under his or her spell. Incidentally, I do not remember ever reaching the bottom of the stairs. What matters the utmost is that I quit smoking afterwards.

Of course, I underwent withdrawals, which were very unpleasant, during which time it was tempting just to pick up a cigarette and start smoking again because by doing so the painful withdrawals would stop, but I wanted desperately to quit. Just about this time my father, who had been a lifelong smoker, had been diagnosed with emphysema, and, after seeing him suffer, I did not want that to happen to me.

After approximately two weeks I felt that the withdrawals had blissfully ceased; but it took me a very long time to get over my craving for a cigarette. My husband and I would go out to dinner frequently because we both worked, oftentimes late hours, and having dinner out was something that we enjoyed doing together. During those days smoking was allowed in restaurants in California, and it would be difficult for me to be in that atmosphere for very long, as I would be tempted by the mere smell of the smoke. Somehow that baby's coffin filled to the brim with those cigarette butts would evoke a vision in my mind intense enough to convince me that this is where smoking could possibly lead me, to a coffin of my own prematurely, and I eventually got over my craving a cigarette and was proud to say that I had joined the ranks of the non-smokers. Sadly, as I was to find out fifteen years later, it was too late.

CHAPTER SIX

After our first meeting with Dr. Harris, he indicated that he wanted me to commence taking chemotherapy immediately. There was a chemo lab in the Fountain Valley Cancer Center where his office was located. Incidentally, Dr. Harris was one of three or four other oncologists in this same office. I'm sure the other oncologists were equally as competent as Dr. Harris was, but I feel extremely blessed to have been referred to this particular oncologist because he was to become one of my mainstays during the months ahead, the first and foremost being my husband Joe.

After our initial consultation Dr. Harris, my husband and I walked back to the chemo lab, where the doctor introduced my husband and me to the small staff of nurses and began to issue his orders that I was to start treatment immediately. This eight-hour session would be my first of twenty-four treatments. I was to attend the Fountain Valley Cancer Center three days a week for a three-day period each week, with one week off to give my body a rest from the intensely aggressive chemotherapy treatments that I was prescribed. This scenario would continue for a period of six months. The first day of the three-day treatment would be for an eight-hour session, and the second and third days would be four hours each. I was told that with this modality of treatment my body would be given a rest for one week; and just about the time I was beginning to recuperate from the chemotherapy treatments of the previous three weeks, the next set of treatments were to begin again. This was the pattern that followed during the next six months.

Before I knew it, I was seated in a chair, my husband sitting beside me, and the lab technician was inserting a needle into a vein in one of my hands so that the combination of drugs that Dr. Harris had prescribed could be given to me intravenously. The entire time went by very slowly and I felt as though I were in a fog.

The lab was a small one, serviced by two lab technicians who were nurses, Joyce and Robert, the supervising nurse. There were maybe seven chairs at the most in the room. Now, these chairs were meant to be comfortable, although they were covered with Naugahyde or vinyl. They did recline, and had armrests and high backs on them, however, so you were able to relax a little bit during treatment, if you were inclined to do so.

That evening after going to bed, I could not go to sleep. When I reported this to the Nurse Robert the following day, he said it was most probably the steroids mixed in with the drugs that kept me awake. Having had no experience whatsoever with what went into a chemo cocktail, I wondered if he was putting me on about the steroids. He was not. At any rate, because I lay there after that first eight-hour session of chemotherapy well into the early morning hours tossing and turning, I got out of bed and went into my office where I did the bulk of my job as a court reporter: transcription, placing telephone calls, doing research, et cetera. There I opened up the computer and wrote a very long e-mail to everybody we knew, telling them about my emotionally wrought day and the events leading up to it. I titled the subject line "Sleepless in Huntington Beach." I thought that very appropriate at the time, Huntington Beach being our place of residence, and, of course, my experiencing absolute insomnia after my first treatment. I had recently seen the movie *Sleepless in Seattle*; thus the title.

CHAPTER SEVEN

Somehow I got through the next two days of chemotherapy. I remember being frightened of the whole scenario, once again not knowing what the future held for me. Fear of the unknown. After reporting to Nurse Robert about my inability to sleep that first night, both Nurse Robert and Nurse Joyce sent me home with some prescriptions for Ambien, which was a sleeping pill, a drug called Kytril that would relieve nausea or vomiting, which are side effects of chemotherapy, and some other drugs which I cannot remember the names of as I write this. I do remember that I was given one of those seven-day pill holders and instructed by one of the nurses regarding just what drugs to take on which day. For me this was unnerving because I have always been a person who rarely even took an aspirin. Nevertheless after having completed my chemotherapy treatment for that day I would begin the regimen of faithfully taking my medicine and my injections of Neupogen and Epogen.

The vials of Neupogen and Epogen were to counteract the low blood count that I was expected to develop from the chemotherapy. The low blood count followed soon thereafter, along with acute anemia. Nurse Robert asked me whether or not I could administer a shot of these drugs to myself every day, and

I thought I would pass out from the mere thought of injecting myself with a needle, let alone having to do it on a daily basis. Of course, there were very explicit instructions given to me along with these vials of Neupogen and Epogen. It just so happened that my husband had been trained while in the service to administer shots to people, so I was in luck because he was more than happy to administer the Neupogen and Epogen to me, and I was ecstatic not to have to do it.

Joe would alternate the shots, Neupogen one day and Epogen the next. These shots made me extremely tired, and I found that I would become overwhelmingly fatigued and would sleep a great deal during the daytime. Nurse Robert had told me to expect this to happen, and not to fight the feeling of fatigue, but to give into it and lie down because my body was in desperate need of the rest in order to assist in my recovery.

Neupogen, in lay terms, is a drug which encourages bone marrow to produce new white blood cells. Epogen is a drug which stimulates the bone marrow to produce new red blood cells. These drugs are essential to a person undergoing chemotherapy because the treatment for cancer, namely chemotherapy, along with destroying the cancer cells, will sometimes have harmful side effects on the body, one of those being destroying the red as well as the white blood cells. Neupogen and Epogen counteract those particular unwanted side effects.

I was tired all of the time, and it seemed that as the days and weeks passed I slept an awful lot during the day as well as at night. I credit my sleeping well at night to Ambien because in the beginning I was experiencing a difficult time getting to sleep, as Nurse Robert told me I would, due to the steroids in my chemo cocktail. I was grateful that I had made the decision to retire from court reporting some eight months prior to the onset of lung cancer because it took every ounce of strength I had to fight this debilitating disease in an attempt to get well again.

After my first three chemotherapy treatments I called Antonio Vargus, my hair stylist, and asked that he cut my hair very short, in anticipation of its falling out during the coming months. Sherry Ross, a good friend and neighbor, drove me to Tony's salon because even at this early stage of the game I did not trust myself behind the wheel. After experiencing my first three treatments of chemotherapy, driving a car somehow just did not feel right. It was as if I didn't have complete control of the situation. I was not as alert as I should be while behind the wheel. It became evident that I had no depth perception, which Nurse Robert later told me was a common side effect of treatment. He said that the drugs were causing the configuration of my eyeballs to change somewhat, and that was the reason for my lack of depth perception.

I was fortunate because I had some friends who were able to drive me to the Cancer Center for my treatments; and most of the time these people would stay there with me until all of the drugs had been absorbed into my system, and then drive me home again. Other times they would drop me off and then return to pick me up after I was finished with my treatment.

I remember one time when Jim Henderson, a good friend whom we had met at church, drove me to my appointment, and he was to return four hours later. Well, for some reason on this particular day Nurse Joyce had set up the IV so that it dripped the drugs into my system somewhat quicker than usual, and I was ready to go home prior to four hours. As it turned out, I ended up waiting in the lobby in the downstairs reception area for about an hour and a half. I called Jim, but he was out and about running errands, as he told me he would be. Those things happen sometimes. I vividly recall that I was especially glad to get home on that day.

The nurses at the lab were extremely nice about allowing the friend or relative who came with one of their patients to stay in the lab to keep the patient company, providing there were extra chairs available, and at that time there usually always were. I was thankful for this because personally it gave me a good deal of support and encouragement to have somebody present whom I was close to.

Beverly Vernon, another very good friend of mine, was very generous with her time, and in the beginning she drove me to a number of my treatments, then drove me back home again. This, of course, was before she began to withdraw from our relationship, as I will explore in the next chapter. Sherry Ross, a friend and neighbor of ours, was kind enough to drive me to and from some of my treatments; Jane Adamson, also a friend and neighbor of ours and whom I worked with as a court reporter, drove me to and from treatments; and last but not least, Jim Henderson drove me a time or two.

CHAPTER EIGHT

Beverly Vernon, a very good friend whom I had gone through court reporting school with, had also retired from her job as a superior court reporter and on occasion would drive me to and from some of my chemotherapy treatments. But Beverly was taking care of an elderly husband who was terminally ill, and she had recently lost a daughter-in-law whom she loved very much to cancer; so it wasn't long before she stopped driving me to my treatments, and eventually fazed out of my life altogether. She had a good deal on her plate, and I believe that she simply couldn't see a close friend stricken with cancer who could possibly die just as her daughter-in-law recently had. At least that's what I would tell myself before I came to the stark realization that, for some reason which I was totally unaware of, she literally wanted me removed from her life entirely. It became apparent that getting her forthcoming single life jump-started was more important to her than what I considered to be our friendship at the time. I would tell myself that she had just gone through a similar situation with her daughter-in-law, whom she was very close to and had driven to chemotherapy treatments, also, and maybe she just needed a break from all of the sickness which was surrounding her, referring to her terminally ill husband, and then there was my having recently been diagnosed with lung cancer.

Beverly, her husband Bill, my husband Joe and I were very close friends for many years. We socialized often and would invite them for weekend visits. The two of them had a boat, and would often invite us to accompany them to Catalina Island for a few days. Then when they retired and moved to Big Bear Lake, a resort community in the mountains outside of the Los Angeles basin, we would drive to this beautiful town nestled away in the San Bernardino Mountains to visit with our friends and to enjoy the clean air and majestic pine trees. In fact, they had fallen in love with Big Bear years earlier when we'd had a second home there, and Joe and I would invite them for a weekend visit.

After they retired to this beautiful mountain community of Big Bear Lake, California, we bought yet another second home just around the corner from where Beverly and Bill lived. We were such close friends that Beverly and I had begun referring to each other as sisters. When we had our hair cut in similar styles people used to tell us that we even looked alike. We would give each other birthday cards and Christmas cards that were specifically for sisters. During a wild evening that we spent together, perhaps after one too many libations, she and I went so far as to prick our fingers in order to draw blood, and then joined our fingers together, as we'd seen done in the movies, leaving us to believe that each of us had the other's blood running through our veins.

This is yet another reason why her terminating what I thought was a thriving friendship between us without an explanation or as much as a goodbye was so devastating to me. It took me a very long period of time to close the door on that phase of my life and open a new one. I finally realized that she must not have been the good friend I thought she was if she could turn her back as easily as she had and walk away from what I perceived to be our friendship which had lasted more than twenty years.

Anticipating the inevitable, Beverly placed her husband in a facility that would care for him, and she began leading a single life, meeting new, single people. Although she did give me a "coming out" party after I had finished my chemotherapy treatments—actually, it was a joint party, also a "coming out" party for her to celebrate her journey into the single life—after the day of the party she drifted farther and farther away until there was no contact between us whatsoever any more.

I mourned losing Beverly as though she were a friend who had died because I knew in my heart that she'd chosen to step out of my life for good. I had not been hurt like that by another human being in many years, and at the time it was very difficult for me to accept, as my emotions were already being stretched to the limit what with having cancer and undergoing chemo-therapy treatment for it, enduring the side effects of the treatment: losing my hair, losing my voice, not knowing if it would return, or even whether or not I would recover from this dreaded disease, experiencing severe neuropathy of my hands and feet, nausea, constipation, incontinence, diarrhea, anemia, and not knowing what was in store for me in the future.

When this happened it broke my heart into very tiny little pieces. I found that I would fall into crying jags for no apparent reason and would cry like a baby at times. One time I was sitting in the dentist's chair having my quarterly cleaning and curettage, and once again the tears began to flow uncontrolla-bly. The hygienist was afraid she had hurt me while cleaning my teeth; so I lied and simply told her that due to the chemo treatments I had undergone in the recent past, my emotions were on the surface and would sometimes run amok.

The hurt I experienced at this time pierced my inner being. It's no wonder I was an emotional wreck. I had lost a person who I thought was one of my dearest friends whom I had known for over twenty years. This was very difficult for me to understand or to accept. We had been so close that I never thought a thing like this could happen.

As compassionate human beings we believe that when we are stricken with a serious illness, those we hold dear will remain close or become even closer to us, but that is not always the case. I have heard other cancer survivors in my cancer support group say that they, too, lost their best friend or somebody dear to them, even family members backed away from them once they were diagnosed with cancer. So apparently what occurred between Beverly and me after I became ill is not so uncommon after all.

The two of us used to joke about living together at the old age home when we were in our golden years. Even if she became a single person by losing her husband, which did eventually happen, I saw no reason why we couldn't still remain friends, but she evidently saw it differently and I was no longer to be a part of her life. It was a rude awakening for me. She did not even notify us of Bill's death, and, therefore, we were unable to pay him our last respects.

It was difficult, but I somehow managed to do what I had to do to get over having lost her friendship. I closed that chapter, opened a new one, and proceeded as best I could to get on with my life. After all, I was now in the ten percentile lung cancer survival group, and I had my whole life ahead of me.

CHAPTER NINE

I had heard all of the horror stories about chemotherapy patients losing their hair, and, of course, I had seen movies in which that happened. The nurses at the lab told me that ninety-nine times out of one hundred patients who undergo chemotherapy will lose their hair, but there was that one percent chance that it wouldn't happen to me. I really was not looking forward to losing my hair. However, it did not take very long before my cherished brown locks began falling out. They were all over my pillow one morning when I awoke. That's when I went to my husband and asked him to "buzz" me.

Off to the garage we went, and there he took the clippers to my already short hair. In a few minutes I looked like a new armed forces recruit might look in boot camp on their first day. My hair still continued to fall out. I would become aware before it happened that it was going to do so because my head would actually ache. I could feel the tiny little hairs freeing themselves from my scalp. Then the next morning the evidence of what had happened during the night would be all over the pillow. That was before I started wearing a head cover to bed, which made an amazing difference in my life.

One morning while I was undergoing a chemotherapy treatment, Nurse Joyce told me that the American Cancer Society had a branch office downstairs on the first floor. I had inquired about whether or not she knew of any support groups that were available to cancer patients in the area. The particular support groups pertaining to lung cancer were all held at night, understandably, because the moderators worked during the day and would volunteer their time after hours. It was just not feasible for me to attend a night session because of my inability to drive and especially to drive at night, so I quickly decided that I'd forego the support group.

I did, however, join a cancer support group through our church after my husband and I retired and relocated back east. I joined this group three months after we arrived in 2001, and have been with this group ever since. I strongly urge anybody undergoing cancer treatment or anyone who is a cancer survivor to join a cancer support group. There is no describing how much you gain from these sessions, and it is all positive.

To quote a beautiful passage that I read which was contained in a pamphlet in my nephrologist's office in Morgantown, West Virginia, while waiting to see her, author unknown: "Just as the beautiful colors of the rainbow have a special meaning: red signifies love; orange, abundance; yellow, happiness; green, hope; indigo, dreams; blue, life; and violet, peace," so do the lives of each one of the survivors in our group. We have all gone through treatment, albeit different types of treatment for different kinds of cancers, but we have that common bond which exists among no others, and it cannot help but bring us close together. These meetings are always comforting and very uplifting, and each one of us seems to gain strength from all the other cancer survivors in our group. A newcomer to the group commented recently on his surprise to see just how uplifting and positive we all are and how pleased he is that he started coming to the meetings.

The volunteers at the American Cancer Society in Fountain Valley, California, did introduce me to a wonderful little catalog that carried a variety of products for cancer patients who had lost their hair, patients who had undergone mastectomies, and so on. I ordered some cotton hats through this catalog; and they, along with scarves, worked very well for me. I did buy a wig, but it was very uncomfortable to wear, most of all because it itched my tender scalp, and so I preferred the cotton hats and scarves. Many of the ladies in my cancer support group have also expressed a distaste for wearing a wig. Of course, at home I didn't wear anything at all on my head, which felt extremely good.

It was strange at first to look in the mirror and see myself with a bald head, not to mention no eyebrows and no eyelashes. They all fell out. In fact, every hair on my body fell out until I was as hairless as I was as the day I was born, hair on a newborn's head being the exception. I had none. To this day the hair has not grown back on my arms nor under my arms, and very little on my legs, but thankfully it's grown back on the rest of my body.

I was especially grateful that it grew back on my head, and when it did it resembled a tight permanent. Today it has a soft, natural curl to it. Before my chemotherapy treatment it was as straight as a pin. The nurses at the chemo lab told me that after treatment it could conceivably grow back any color that it had ever been during my lifetime. So because I had been a redhead as a baby, I was hoping it would grow back red because I've always admired reddish/auburn hair. But it grew back my natural color, dark brown, and I was so happy to have hair again that what color it was didn't really matter. At least I had hair.

I felt conspicuous because of my hair situation, or lack thereof, so I didn't venture out very often except to go to the doctor and to my chemotherapy treatments. Sometime after my hair began to grow back somewhat and I was blessed with a slight covering of fuzzy "frog hair" on my scalp, my confidence began to return. It was on one of Joe's days off during this time that we decided to go for a ride. While we were out he decided to go into a Sports Mart so he could pick up something that he needed. Joe had been telling me ever since my hair fell out how good I looked bald, how perfectly my head was shaped, and that if our roles were reversed and he had been the one undergoing treatment for cancer and had lost all of his hair, that he would look awful because of the odd shape of his skull and all the scars that he had on his head. So on this particular day, with his prodding and my self-confidence bursting at the seams, I ventured out in the afternoon with no head covering. My head resembled that of a newborn's.

Now, keep in mind that we lived in Southern California where almost anything goes. We had even seen people who had shaved their heads purposely and then had their bald heads tattooed in order to make a fashion statement. So with my legitimate reason for having no hair, I should have blended right in and there should not have been a problem. Right? Wrong.

I was in one of the aisles at the Sports Mart, thinking I looked pretty good, full of poise and confidence. I was standing there observing a display when I heard someone say, "Would you look at her. People like that should know better than to go out in public." I looked up and saw a man and a woman staring at me, making faces and smacking their lips, "Tch-tch," and I quickly realized that I was the brunt of their jibes. Talk about having your confidence bubble deflated. I know I shouldn't have let their actions get to me, I should have considered the source; but I was immediately devastated. My husband also observed this taking place, and he asked them if there was a problem, but naturally they made no response; and we left the store within a short time after that.

They say that sometimes children can be cruel. I say adults can be just as cruel as children, and the adults should know better.

CHAPTER TEN

I could not escape losing my hair, but I began to think that I was going to be one of the blessed patients who go through chemotherapy without becoming sick to my stomach. The reason I felt this way was because I'd gone for six weeks without becoming ill. So here I was a month and a half into my chemotherapy treatment thinking this was going to be a breeze, with the exception of losing all my hair. It wasn't until approximately between my second and third series of treatments that I began to feel nauseous. So that euphoric feeling that I was going to escape becoming sick to my stomach did not last very long at all. Oh, I was taking the Kytril faithfully, and they would also insert something into the chemo cocktail which was supposed to keep me from getting sick to my stomach, but eventually even that didn't help and I was not able to hold much of anything down.

I had no appetite, but I was aware that I had to eat to keep up my strength. Along with having to attend work daily, my husband took over the kitchen duties as well as the household duties after I'd become ill. I tried as hard as I could to eat what Joe cooked for me. The reason he took over these chores is because I was simply too weak to do them. Honestly, I was so wrought with fatigue because of the anemia I was experiencing that I could barely lift a finger during this time.

Joe is a good cook, as most men are, and he always fixed something delicious and nourishing or whatever it was that I happened to be craving. I would crave different foods sometimes, such as chili, pasta and shrimp, and even Fritos corn chips. The chili and Fritos were unusual cravings in that we never had these items in our cupboards, unless we were about to have a party or a bar-b-que. But rarely would either of these items cross my lips, and here I was craving them like a pregnant woman craves pickles and ice cream. The chemo must have been depleting the sodium from my body. Why else would I have been craving some of these sodium-enriched foods?

Under normal circumstances I would have eaten every single bite of a meal that Joe fixed. The sight and the smell of food, however, was extremely distasteful to me. I was lucky if I could take two or three bites of the meals he would prepare, and then afterwards I would have to leave the table and go straight to our bedroom. Here I would lie quietly on the bed to gain solace where only the light from the radio would be illuminating the room. I would have the radio tuned to a classical music station which was broadcasting from the University of California campus at Long Beach, and it would be on very softly. During my treatment I became unable to endure bright light and loud sounds, the television, for example, which would be loud enough when it was on so that my hearing-impaired husband could enjoy it. Even the sunlight as seen from the inside of the house was difficult to bear. Other cancer survivors in my cancer support group have indicated that they felt the same way while they were undergoing their treatment; so the inability to endure bright light and loud sounds must be a prevalent side effect of chemotherapy.

Our bedroom became my refuge, and I spent many hours there contemplating my situation, talking to God, telling Him that if it's His will that I do not survive these treatments, that I was ready to come home. There were times when I was wrought with such hopelessness that I could not help but feel that this was a very real possibility. I also asked Him often to take me into His arms and to hold me; and I told Him how much I needed Him to comfort me and to give me the strength I needed to get through the coming months. It may have been a one-sided conversation, but my faith was victorious, and I know He heard me talking to Him because I was to draw on the strength that He gave me many times in the months to come.

I was not able to keep solid food down, so I tried drinking some Ensure because it contained many vitamins and lots of calories and was very nourishing, but I could not endure very many of those meals. With apologies to the company who makes the product, it simply did not taste good to me. I'm certain that if I drank some Ensure today I would enjoy the taste; however, I most certainly don't need the extra calories today the way I did then. What seemed to agree with me was chicken noodle soup accompanied by crackers or toast. That was soothing and for some reason it tasted exceptionally good, plus I was able to keep it down. Also, it was easy to fix and I didn't have to expend very much energy to do so. Just add water and the soup mixture into a bowl, pop it into the microwave, and in two or three minutes you have a very satisfying bowl of soup. Early on in my treatment I became anemic, and my blood count became so low that I could barely drag myself around the house from chair to chair without having to stand there and catch my breath because I was panting as though I'd run a mile. So being able to fix a nourishing and tasty lunch in a matter of minutes was very much appreciated by me.

I was not the type of person to sit in front of a television set during the day, or at night, for that matter, unless it was a good movie, but because my physical activity was limited and due to fatigue caused by the anemia, my daily routine became watching television while I had lunch, then sitting there to watch some of the other daytime programs. I would also call Joe at work to say hello and let him know how I was doing, and that I had eaten lunch because he was concerned that I wasn't getting enough nourishment. During this time I discovered that there's an awful lot of trash being televised. We did not have cable or the satellite hooked up to our television in the living room. I spent most of my days there and not in our family room where we did have satellite capability because the living room was much closer to the kitchen, our bedroom and the bathrooms. I was limited to the local channels, which suited me just fine. It passed the time during the day while Joe was at work.

There's almost nothing more I enjoy than reading a good book, but I could not do so because I was unable to concentrate on one paragraph, let alone read an entire book. Even reading a sentence over more than once was of no use; I simply could not retain what was written on the page before me. My mind was somehow befuddled because of the drugs that were being administered to me in the chemotherapy cocktails and I could not concentrate. We in our cancer support group refer to this condition as "chemo brain," and almost all of us occasionally experience "chemo brain" today, many years after treatment. It can manifest itself in different ways. As an example, some people will start a sentence and be unable to finish it because they've forgotten what they started to say. You tend to write things down so as not to forget what you need to do on a certain day. I thought I was the only person this was happening to until I learned at a cancer support group meeting that other members of the group experienced this problem as well. Then I didn't feel so bad because I wasn't alone. This seemed to be a common occurrence among everyone.

One morning I had an appointment to see Dr. Harris for lab work which would consist of his nurse drawing my blood and running it through the machine they had on the premises to see what my readings were. In this way they could tell whether or not I was anemic, what my creatinine level was, and in general how I was responding to the chemotherapy treatment. I was going to drive myself to the Cancer Center on this particular morning. While I was getting ready to go, I was overcome with nausea, and was on the bathroom floor vomiting into the toilet. Vomiting, of course, is another side effect of the chemotherapy. I called Joe at work to tell him what was happening, and that I didn't think I'd be able to drive myself to see Dr. Harris. I had become very ill and was extremely weak. He drove home from work to pick me up and take me to my appointment.

When I saw the doctor, I told him what had happened. He ordered the lab work taken, and, of course, the results confirmed that my red blood count was extremely low. I was even more anemic than I had been when they had taken any prior lab work.

Anemia is a shortage of red blood cells or a protein found in them (hemoglobin). The red blood cells carry oxygen throughout the body. Symptoms of anemia may include: Shortness of breath, severe fatigue (feeling tired all the time), pale skin, feeling cold, confusion or loss of concentration, and dizziness or fainting. I was given iron injections periodically for the anemia during the six months of my treatment.

My blood was monitored once or twice a week, even during the weeks I wasn't receiving chemotherapy treatments, and this continued to be the case after my treatments ceased. Oftentimes I was given iron shots because my blood count was below normal. These shots would make me feel a little better, but only for a short period of time, then the overwhelming fatigue would return. To this day I still have a shadow of the bruising on my left hip from all of those iron shots that I was administered. I find that hard to believe myself, but it's true.

After Joe got home that morning he drove me to Dr. Harris's office. Dr. Harris called next door to the Infusion Center, told them we were on our way over, that he wanted me to have a blood transfusion immediately, for them to have everything ready by the time we got there, and the three of us walked over there together.

This was the first of three blood transfusions that I was administered during the six-month period of my treatment. It was a very frightening experience. Fear of the unknown and all of that. I experienced an emotional roller coaster each time I sat in the chair and the nurse inserted the needle into my vein. Naturally my first thought was of the possibility of my contracting the AIDS virus through the blood transfusions. But apparently they had their screening procedures pretty well down pat by this time in 1999, and I was assured that I would be all right, not to worry. Just the same, I did my share of worrying.

During a blood transfusion whole blood or blood component is introduced directly into the bloodstream via a needle or catheter placed in the vein. All three times that I received a blood transfusion it was as cold as ice as it entered my vein, thus it was extremely painful. I have a low tolerance for pain, and that may explain my feeling the way I did. As uncomfortable as it was, each time I seemed to get through it all right.

I recollect the nurse at least once telling me that the blood she was administering to me had been warmed up, but once it entered my bloodstream, I had serious doubts about just how long it had been kept on the warming apparatus. In fact, some patients in this very small lab who were also receiving blood transfusions were sitting there with small heaters plugged into the wall, enjoying the heat that they were transmitting. I assume this was to keep them warm while they underwent this grueling (in my opinion) procedure.

The blood transfusions really did help alleviate my anemia and I began to feel better after each one, but that initial burst of energy was short-lived and would be a mere pleasant memory once I began treatment again because the anemia would return with a great intensity.

Three months into my treatments while I was at one of my weekly visits with Dr. Harris, he informed me that the recent CT scan had revealed that the tumors on my lung and liver were gone. I was elated. Of course, the first thought that came to mind was, Hallelujah! I don't have to continue with chemotherapy; I'm cured. Well, not so. When I asked Dr. Harris if I could stop attending the chemo lab to receive my treatments, he said no. As pleased as he was that the tumors were gone and that the treatment he'd prescribed appeared to be working perfectly, he proceeded to tell me that there could be some more cancer cells floating around inside my body, and that I needed to finish my prescribed modality of treatment to be sure that all of the cells were eliminated. He likened this to baking a cake and he said that unless you include all of the ingredients in the cake mix, the cake will not be a success. In other words, if you leave an important part out, such as the baking soda, the cake will not rise. That put it into perspective for me, and I forged on in my treatments.

CHAPTER ELEVEN

One day a woman who used to work for my husband and whom I was acquainted with, also, came to his place of work to visit some of her friends. She was told about my having cancer and the nausea that I had been experiencing. She quickly told Joe that he should get me some marijuana because she'd heard that it would help the nausea. I kid you not. This lovely lady's name was Sammi Schultz. And while I'm sure she meant well, Joe just laughed at her suggestion and said that it was, of course, out of the question, not to mention that, even if he knew where to go and what to do to get it, he wouldn't put his job in jeopardy. Sammi was in her seventies at this time, cute as a button, and she could have passed for fifty-something easily. She said it wasn't a problem, that she would get it for me. Needless to say, there was no marijuana purchased, and I got along just fine without it. Well, as fine as could be expected, anyway.

Once the nausea began, however, it seemed as though that feeling of impending illness was always there lurking in the background ready to strike again. And strike again it did, many times over. It became most prevalent after I'd had a three-day chemotherapy session. Sometimes the nausea would occur several days after my treatment when I would least expect it, but once it started I could always count on getting sick to my stomach. It's no wonder I became anemic once the nausea began; I couldn't hold any food, solids or liquids, down whatsoever for very long. I lost twenty-five pounds during this period of time.

Other side effects of the chemotherapy were constipation, diarrhea, and at times incontinence. I would attempt to pass gas, and ooops! "liquid gas" would escape from my body. What a surprise that would be. Thank goodness this particular malady only lasted for a short period of time. But it was very real. After the first surprise that nature bestowed upon me, I attempted not passing gas, or doing so only while sitting on the commode.

I was encouraged by the nurses at the chemo lab to drink lots of water, as much as I could stand to drink, hopefully to flush the drugs through and out of my system. They also suggested I keep hard candies available to moisten my dry mouth. Water began to taste metallic, almost exactly like the chemicals in the chemo itself, and it was difficult for me to drink a lot of it. When I told this to Nurse Robert, he said that some of their patients find that it's a lot more tolerable to drink the carbonated, flavored waters, and it would be good if I would try to do this. I stocked up on different flavors of this beverage, and drank it 'til the cows came home. Nurse Robert was right, it was more tolerable, and I always had a glass of carbonated, flavored ice water nearby so that I could force myself to drink at least a quart a day. Unfortunately I no longer can look at a bottle of that flavored, carbonated water without gagging. I drank so much of it during my treatment that eventually I could taste the chemicals from the chemotherapy in this water, also, and the metallic smell of the chemicals is what mysteriously permeates the air when I get in the same aisle at the supermarket with some of those bottles today. I'm sure it's psychosematic, but nevertheless that's what happens to me.

Another side effect of the chemotherapy that I experienced and still experience today is peripheral neuropathy of my hands and feet, which *Dorland's Illustrated Medical Dictionary 27th Edition* defines as "A general term denoting functional disturbances and/or pathological changes in the peripheral nervous system." Your fingers and toes may feel numb, tingle, burn or hurt. Peripheral neuropathy may or may not go away. At first the symptoms were so severe that I could not write legibly; I had to print instead of writing, slowly and carefully I might add, in order for it to be legible. I definitely could not recognize my own handwriting during this period of time.

As for my feet, I could barely feel them for they were so numb. It was like experiencing nonstop pins and needles. In fact, that feeling in my feet traveled part of the way up my legs so that it felt as though I were walking on wooden stumps, not my own feet or legs.

When I asked Dr. Harris about this symptom and how long he thought it would last, he said that it would last a long time, he had no way of knowing just how long. While this condition has improved, it is still present today in both my hands and my feet, although it's not as prevalent as it was in the beginning. It is more predominant in my feet. I'm unable to wear two-inch heels anymore because the lack of feeling in my feet causes me to be less able to keep my balance; and I find myself frequently twisting my ankles if I do try to wear shoes with even the slightest heel.

This condition was evidenced recently by my having gone barefoot on our back deck and not being aware that I'd stepped on a wood splinter which became lodged in my left foot. Now, the splinter was approximately three quarters of an inch long, so it was a splinter to be reckoned with. I became aware of this after walking on it for a few days; and then while I was taking a hot Jacuzzi bath, enjoying the sensation of the pulsing jets on my feet, I finally began to experience some soreness in my left foot. I asked my husband to check it out, and when he did and he told me what it was, I asked him to remove it. After he did so, I felt much better.

Peripheral neuropathy is a common side effect of chemotherapy. A friend in my cancer support group has been out of treatment for twenty-five years now, and she still experiences numbness and tingling in her hands and feet. Other survivors in our group also experience the same symptoms in their feet and hands many years after their treatment.

Thrombocytopenia: "A decrease in the number of blood platelets," as defined by *Dorland's Illustrated Medical Dictionary 27th Edition*, resulted in my having ecchymosis. Ecchymosis is "a small hemorrhagic spot, larger than a petechia (a pinpoint, non-raised perfectly round, purplish red spot caused by intradermal or submucous hemorrhage), in the skin or mucous membrane forming a nonelevated, rounded or irregular, blue or purplish patch," also as defined by *Dorland's Illustrated Medical Dictionary 27th Edition*. In other words, after commencing chemotherapy treatments I began to bruise very easily. This symptom does not exist today to the extent that it did when I was undergoing treatment, but I do bruise more easily now from the slightest bump than I ever did before I began to undergo treatment.

Also, my immune system is not as strong as it was before I was stricken with lung cancer and the subsequent treatment that I received for it. The chemotherapy dealt my immune system a very heavy blow, and because of that if I'm around somebody with a cold, I can almost count on coming down with it. Consequently I try the best I can to avoid being around people who are ill. I have had more colds and viruses since I finished with treatment than I've ever had in my lifetime. It's very frustrating because I was always essentially a healthy person. If I had one cold a year, that was a lot. I understand the reason why I become ill more often now, but it's still another frustrating side effect of treatment.

CHAPTER TWELVE

One of the most uncomfortable side effects of my having lung cancer was losing my voice. This lasted approximately eight or nine months, although at the time it felt like much longer. The tumor on my lung was positioned resting against the recurrent laryngeal nerve for a long period of time, long enough for it to impact that nerve severely, thus causing me to lose my voice. *Dorland's Illustrated Medical Dictionary 27th Edition* defines recurrent as "running back or towards the source," and laryngeal is defined as "of or pertaining to the larynx." The recurrent laryngeal nerve is attached to the larynx, which is defined by *Dorland's* as "the essential sphincter guarding the entrance into the trachea and functioning secondarily as the organ of voice." In other words, the voice box.

I was completely devastated when I lost my voice, especially after I was told by Dr. Johnson, my general practitioner, Dr. Harris, my oncologist, and Dr. Fuller, my E.N.T., ear, nose and throat doctor whom I treated with for many months, that my voice may never return. Dr. Johnson explained to me that sometimes this nerve has been known to repair itself, and that if it did so in my case, it would take a very long time for it to regenerate because the nerve was very lengthy, but for me not to count on that happening because there were no guarantees that it would regenerate. I reluctantly became more or less resigned to being speechless for the rest of my life. But I knew that would not be the end of the world. After all, there were many more people who had worse maladies than not being able to speak.

However, this did present an interesting problem at home. Since my husband is hearing impaired and sometimes wears hearing aides and since I could not talk above a mere whisper, we had to communicate mostly by my writing him notes. At first he was wearing his hearing aides all the time in order to hear what I had to say to him via my whispering, but then he got a terrible ear infection and had to stop wearing them. In fact, Joe treated with Dr. Fuller, my E.N.T. doctor, for a few visits until his ear infection cleared up.

Having been faced with the possibility of going through life without being able to speak opened a whole new area of anxiety and hopelessness within me. Since I did not have a voice, I could not communicate my feelings and thoughts to anyone about what I was undergoing with the chemotherapy, what I was feeling, what my fears were, what I hoped would come of all of this. My innermost thoughts. I decided when I got better that I would take a course in sign language at our local community college, and I intended to encourage Joe to do the same; therefore, some day we would be able to communicate more easily with one another through sign. Luckily with the passage of time it wasn't necessary that we do so because my voice did eventually return. I for one am extremely pleased about that. It's so much nicer to be able to communicate verbally with everyone.

It may sound silly, but when I lost my voice there were times when I used to wonder what would happen if I were to find myself in a situation where I really needed it, such as if I were being attacked in a mall parking lot or an underground parking garage, or what if somebody attempted to rob me. As we're all aware, these events do happen every day in our metropolitan areas and some of our rural areas, as well. I know that I could not scream for help because I tried doing so when this thought came to mind, and no sound escaped my throat. I could not even laugh out loud. Imagine for just a minute what it feels like not to be able to hear yourself laugh. On the brighter side, I told myself that I'd get a loud whistle to wear around my neck, and that should suffice to put my mind at ease because I could blow the whistle if I were ever accosted. When I did so hopefully it would bring help, or with some luck the perpetrator would be so shocked that he would run for the hills.

It's really not surprising that I would entertain thoughts such as these because, after all, I was a court reporter for twenty-two years and spent an awful lot of time in court transcribing preliminary hearings and criminal trials, and my husband had been in law enforcement for nine years and did not hesitate to share some of his experiences and those of his fellow officers with me. So I was far from being naive about the subject, and I knew the threat of something like that happening to me or to anyone, for that matter, was very real.

One day when Joe came home from work I told him about a thought that had occurred to me that day. I said that it would be interesting for me to attempt to get on one of those hair-raising rides at Disneyland which forces men and women as well as children to scream their heads off because I was unable to scream above a whisper. I believe that because he thought my voice would return to me one day, he sort of brushed that thought aside and replaced it with another more pleasant thought, or it could just be that he tried to take my mind off of such dreadful issues by offering to give me a back massage, which he did frequently during this period of time, and which I always welcomed.

My voice finally returned approximately eight or nine months after it disappeared. Believe me, that was cause for celebration! Our prayers and the prayers of family members and friends were answered. I could then pick up the telephone once more and say, "Hello" without having to knock twice to let the caller know somebody was on the line after picking up the receiver, not to mention the fact that I could hold a genuine conversation with my husband and friends once again. I could finally convey all the thoughts that I had kept bottled up inside of me for such a long period of time. Yes, I had a lot to talk about, and it felt so good to be able to communicate verbally once again. When something like this happens, one becomes aware of all the everyday activities in our lives that we seem to take for granted. What a God-given gift it is being able to speak.

CHAPTER THIRTEEN

A few months later I joined a choir called the Celebration of Life Singers whose members had to be either cancer survivors or caregivers to either a spouse or loved one who had cancer. We performed at cancer support group functions, retirement homes, hospitals, and the like. At a practice session during the holiday season one of our members said that a group who was going to perform at her church Christmas party had to cancel, and she asked if any of us would like to volunteer to sing a few Christmas carols. Four of us, myself included, raised our hands. I honestly don't know what possessed me to do this because I've always shied away from speaking in front of an audience, let alone singing, but a few nights later I found myself on a stage in front of a considerably large group of men and women, my knees literally knocking together because I was so nervous, singing soprano no less. Now, mind you, I'm an alto, but I was so confused because the person standing next to me, who was also an alto, was singing harmony. Harmony! How could she do that to me? I guess I expected her to be singing alto along with me, and, boy, did her singing harmony throw me for a loop. Well, there I was singing soprano for the first time in my very short-lived singing career. Luckily our regular pianist was able to be present, and I believe that we all felt more comfortable and were able to give a better performance by having her there.

I thoroughly enjoyed the time I spent with the Celebration of Life Singers. It was one of the best experiences in my entire lifetime. I looked forward to our practice sessions with such enthusiasm. I would spend hours practicing singing at home, either to the sheet music we had been given, or to the cassette tapes of some of the songs we were learning. These cassette tapes would consist of piano music, and I would sing along as though I were at a real practice session being accompanied by a live pianist. Singing turned out to be one of the most rewarding gifts I could have ever received. I felt as though I were praising God by using the voice He had chosen to give back to me.

CHAPTER FOURTEEN

I had always, before contracting lung cancer, been a rather healthy person, full of boundless energy. All of my adult life I had been very independent. I left home at the tender age of eighteen and was on my own until I met and married my husband at age twenty-seven. You could describe me as a loner. Even after getting married I didn't depend on my husband, mainly because he was still in the U.S. Navy and was away from home an awful lot of the time. At the time that he got out of the service and we moved from San Francisco to Huntington Beach in Southern California, it was a tremendous adjustment for the both of us. Joe began working the graveyard shift, and I was more or less on my own again, taking care of our apartment, attending court reporting school eventually, and just basically taking care of myself. So when I became anemic and was not able to function as a normal person, it was extremely debilitating, and I felt more helpless than I had ever felt in my entire life, not being able to run a vacuum cleaner or do the mundane chores that needed to be done around the house. I simply did not have the energy to lift a finger to do it. Each day it was an effort on my part just to get out of bed, have some breakfast, and get ready for the day. Each movement I made seemed to take all the energy I could muster. For example, getting up from the table and walking to the sink, which was no more than four feet away, would have me gasping for air and I would need to sit down and rest.

One afternoon Robin Moore, a woman in our circle of friends whom I had really never been particularly close to, came to pay me a visit. She had driven up from her new home in the country to visit some mutual friends of ours, Mary and Dennis Hart who lived across the street from us. Joe and I had also been invited to attend the bar-b-que that the Harts were giving, as well as our friends Sheila and Victor Ross, who lived three houses down from the Harts. I stayed home and rested, as I was much too weak to attend the bar-b-que. Joe, Dennis and Robin's late husband Neil had gone on a number of deep-sea fishing trips together, and our mutual friendship went back many years.

Robin, having heard about my illness, walked across the street during this time to pay me a visit. She said that she was sorry I had been unable to attend the bar-b-que, that she had been looking forward to seeing me. During her visit she extended an invitation to come visit her in the country; she said she thought it would be good for me to get out of the house for a few days, and that a change of scenery might be just what I needed. I agreed that it was a good idea. Robin said she would be back to pick me up the next day. I had confided to her that I felt terrible that I was unable to do much picking up around the house, and asked her to overlook the untidy state that the house was in. She said that she was going to come by to get me up at a certain time in the morning, and that she was going to proceed to vacuum and do some dusting for me, and that we would leave for the country afterwards. Even though the dust bunnies were driving me crazy by this time, I, of course, protested about her doing the housework, but she insisted that it was something she wanted to do for me.

What Robin proceeded to do that Monday morning turned out to be the most wonderful gift, one that I never expected from this individual. I shall never forget the kindness that she extended to me at this very low point in my life.

May I take this opportunity to say thank you, Robin. You will never know just what your helping me that day meant to me. It was genuinely the perfect gift.

Easter Sunday of 1999 another friend, Janine Mason, paid us a visit. She brought us a very nice home-cooked dinner, ham, sweet potatoes and all the trimmings. That was an additional pleasant surprise that occurred which was very much appreciated by my husband and myself. Janine stayed and visited with me for a while, and I was so glad that she did so because, although we were the best of friends, she had a very demanding full-time job, and we saw very little of one another. Before I became ill, we would get together on a weekend evening and go out to dinner with her and her husband Jack. After I became ill understandably Joe and I were not able to spend much time visiting with friends.

The reason I haven't mentioned family during this period of time is because my side of the family was living in Northern California near the Oregon border, approximately an eight- to ten-hour drive from our home in Huntington Beach, and Joe's side of the family was spread out across the United States, most of them residing back east. So there were no family members paying us visits as it was geographically inconvenient.

Easter Sunday in 1999 brought another surprise. When Joe went out for the Sunday paper, he came back in with a cute little Easter basket filled with some chocolate eggs and an adorable little Easter bunny. There was no card, so I didn't know who it came from at first. After some clever detective work on my part, however, I arrived at the conclusion that Patty Chapman had dropped it off for me. Patty and Doug Chapman were a very nice couple whom we had met at church. We used to sit in the pew behind them. Being the creatures of habit that we are, it was always the same pew every Sunday. In fact, Patty kept herself very busy sending me a get-well card almost every single day during the time I was sick; and it did wonders for my mental well-being. I found myself looking forward to going to the garage each day and collecting the mail after it was delivered through the mail slot in our garage door because there would inevitably be a get-well card waiting there for me from Patty. The cheerful cards that she sent were very uplifting.

CHAPTER FIFTEEN

By far the worst side effect of my treatment is chronic renal failure, commonly known as kidney disease, chronic being defined by *Dorland's Illustrated 27th Edition Medical Dictionary* as "persisting over a long period of time." The kidneys filter the blood to remove waste that is then removed out of the body in urine. Kidneys that are not working properly cannot filter out the waste. This waste can build up inside your body and make you feel sick.

During one of my follow-up visits after having completed chemotherapy, I asked Dr. Harris, my oncologist, if he would give me a referral to a nephrologist because while doing research on the Internet about cancer and its modality of treatment with chemotherapy, I had discovered that one of the many side effects of chemotherapy is that it can harm the kidneys. Carrie Williams, a dear friend of mine in California who had breast cancer ten years earlier, had told me that she now was being treated for a heart problem, which was also one of the many side effects of chemotherapy. I wanted to be certain that I was experiencing none of the side effects I had read about, and that's why I asked Dr. Harris for a referral to a nephrologist.

Dr. Harris referred me to Dr. Sandburg, who was located in the same medical facility as he was.

After a plethora of very extensive tests ordered by Dr. Sandburg, it was discovered that the chemotherapy had completely destroyed two thirds of my kidney function. As I had feared, the chemotherapy had affected my kidneys. Consequently, in order for me to stay relatively healthy and not to end up on dialysis some day in the future or, worse, to have my heart literally stop beating due to an excess of potassium in my bloodstream, potassium levels being regulated by the kidneys, I must follow a very strict renal diet.

This means that I have to limit my intake of sodium, protein and potassium, which means I have to measure and to weigh all food portions in order to get the proper daily intake necessary, and not too much of the three above-mentioned categories, most especially too much potassium. Having too much potassium in a person's system who has chronic kidney disease is without a doubt a silent killer.

This way of life has become second nature to me after much struggling with it. It becomes ever so much easier, however, to follow my renal diet and to deal with the new lifestyle that I am following because of it when it is viewed as a matter of life and death, which in my case it is.

Promptly after finishing the tests and after those results were provided to Dr. Sandburg, he immediately called me at home about 7:00 p.m. one evening to inform me that my potassium reading was extremely high, well into the danger level, and he wanted me to go to the pharmacy in the Cancer Center in Fountain Valley immediately to purchase some medicine which would counteract this high reading. He knew for certain that they had the drug in stock, and didn't want to take the chance that my pharmacy might have to order it. It was a unique drug used specifically by patients with renal failure; so it most definitely would be in stock at the Cancer Center's pharmacy.

This drug is a foul-tasting liquid medicine called Sodium Polystyrene Sulfonate. Of course, I took Dr. Sandburg's advice, purchased the medicine, and proceeded to drink it right away, doing my best not to gag on it as it went down. I saw Dr. Sandburg very soon after this occurred, had lab work performed again, and he informed me that my potassium reading had indeed gone down, which he was pleased to see happen.

It was during this visit that I was told by Dr. Sandburg that there is no warning whatsoever when a person is absorbing too much potassium into their system. To drive the seriousness of the matter home, he told me that the heart just stops beating, and you will die. Therefore, staying on my renal diet is a small price to pay for me to stay relatively healthy and to avoid having to go on dialysis, not to mention having my heart stop beating unexpectedly one day. An event such as that could almost certainly ruin your day.

After completing my chemotherapy treatments, I was given a Certificate of Completion, a kind, congratulatory gesture which Nurse Diane and Nurse Robert always did to make their patients feel special. Afterwards I underwent CT scans on a regular basis which felt like monthly, although in reality it was every three months, and regular once-a-week visits to Dr. Harris for lab work. They were keeping a close eye on my anemia, and I was receiving iron shots regularly.

During a follow-up visit after one of those CT scans Dr. Harris told me that the tumors had not returned, that I appeared to be cancer-free, and asked me how I was feeling. He was a very personable and caring doctor. I replied that I felt like a million dollars, thanks to him. He insisted that he did nothing that the man upstairs didn't have him do. I was quick to reply that I had many family members and friends praying for me during this period of time. Even some monks in a monastery in Italy were praying for me (a friend of mine knew one of the monks and had told him of my illness), and I told Dr. Harris that this surely couldn't have hurt, either. Then Dr. Harris told me that I really should be feeling like a million dollars, emphasis on "should," because only ten per cent of patients with my type of cancer survive. Of course, I felt as though I were on cloud nine after that. I thank God every day for giving me another chance, and I pray that I'm living my life to His expectations.

Sometimes when a person has been as blessed as I feel that I have been, that person experiences the need to give back to the community. My husband and I have become involved in volunteer work at our church, and doing so has been more rewarding than I could have imagined it would be. Not only that, but we've met and become friends with some very warm, caring people while doing our volunteer work.

CHAPTER SIXTEEN

Presently I'm under the care of Dr. Katherine Martin, a highly respected and competent nephrologist at West Virginia University Hospital in Morgantown, West Virginia. I see Dr. Martin every four or five months, unless a problem surfaces in my lab work, then she will have me return sooner. After she treats me for the problem and it's resolved, she'll have me resume my regular schedule of visits every four to five months. Since I've been going to her the results of my lab work have been relatively unwavering, which means that my following the renal diet to the letter is paying off.

All of my lab results are elevated for a person who does not have chronic kidney disease, but they are in the normal range for me, a person with chronic kidney disease; and as long as they stay within those numbers which are normal for me and do not go any higher, I have been told that I will avoid having to go on dialysis. I cannot reiterate enough that I feel that my following the renal diet is a small price to pay in order to refrain from having to go on dialysis, not to mention avoiding the Grim Reaper because of an extremely high potassium level.

I am grateful to my family members and friends who have been considerate enough to accommodate me with regard to fixing food a certain way when Joe and I have been invited to their homes for dinner. However, I cannot expect family or friends to continue to be considerate of my dietary needs; therefore, I have devised a system that works very well when we're invited to someone's home for a celebration, be it a birthday, Easter, Christmas, etc. I've purchased some little plastic containers with divided compartments. In those containers I will put the food that I've cooked and am able to consume, and then I will take that with me. I can make up six or seven of these at a time and freeze them until I need one. And if we go away for a few days to, say, our relatives in Cleveland, for example, I'll take however many of those dinners I need, and whatever I want to have for lunches. No fuss, no muss. Breakfast is easy. It's cereal, fruit and one half cup of milk. Of course, I can only eat certain cereals and fruits, so I will always bring along whatever it is that I'm allowed to have. I worked on devising this system after some exceptionally rude awakenings, shall we say, rude awakenings on my part.

When we moved back east and began to be invited to participate in our relatives' get-togethers, celebrations such as birthdays, graduations, dinners, etc., I would attend these events along with my husband, going under the delusive assumption that surely I would find something to eat at the event, maybe fruit, bread, cheese, or fresh vegetables. I thought there would be something there that I'm allowed to have. How naive of me. First of all, we are not in California any longer where a variety of the aforementioned foods would be offered as a matter of course, and it didn't take long to realize that fruit, cheese, and fresh vegetables are not high-priority items in our new environment the way they were in our old environment. That includes restaurants and delicatessens as well as private homes.

When we go out to eat it's very disappointing to discover that there is not one thing on the menu that I am allowed in the way of an entree. This has happened to me more times than I can count. What I have done in those cases is I've ordered toast and butter because I am allowed to have that. On one occasion in particular when we stopped for lunch, I hadn't had any breakfast and I was very hungry, so I had a second order of toast and butter. Finding yourself in this situation can be extremely frustrating.

Shortly after being diagnosed with chronic renal failure and soon after I had begun to follow the renal diet, Joe and I were visiting in Northern California where my family lives. This is before we moved to the East Coast. During this particular visit we were looking at a piece of property that we may have been interested in purchasing, and were out and about with a cousin of mine who was going to do some work for us on this property, if we had decided to purchase it. It was lunchtime, and because there were not very many restaurants to choose from in this particular area, we stopped at a deli that my cousin said would be good. I was hoping that I could find something to eat there which is compatible with my renal diet. As it turns out, there was not one thing in the deli case nor anywhere on the shelves that I was allowed to have.

I must have looked awfully bewildered as I stood there waiting for Joe and my cousin to place their sandwich orders because the woman behind the counter asked if there was something that she could get for me. I said no, with somewhat of a catch in my throat, that there was nothing displayed in the deli case that I could have. I also mentioned that I'd recently been put on a special diet because of a medical condition. She kindly asked if I could have vegetables, and when I said I could have some of them, she went in the back, and when she returned she said she had a tomato and some lettuce, and that she would be only too glad to fix it for me. I was so grateful for this simple act of kindness that I said that would be fine. After getting home and studying my renal diet a lot closer, I realized that tomatoes are very high in potassium; so since that experience I've limited my intake of that vegetable, as much as I enjoy having them.

I remember one Sunday morning before we left California when we took some relatives who were visiting us out to a champagne brunch, which was a very popular pastime on Sundays. When we arrived at the restaurant my husband and I were surprised to learn that this particular establishment that we had patronized on Sundays many times in the past had ceased serving their Sunday brunch buffet style, which, of course, would have given us many wonderful choices, including that of fresh fruits and vegetables, fresh breads, cheeses and the like, foods that I was allowed. Instead we had to order off of the menu. I had to scrutinize the menu, and upon doing so I came up with something I could have: a broiled artichoke. I dearly love artichokes, so I ordered that for brunch, and it was extremely delicious.

Our "salad" on this particular Sunday morning consisted of flowers, edible flowers. You should have seen the looks on our relatives' faces when they asked what the flowers were doing on everyone's plate and we told them that was our salad and we were to eat them, which Joe and I proceeded to do. I think I ate one just to prove that what we said was true. I don't honestly know if edible flowers are included in my renal diet. We knew this was the proper procedure, however, because we'd been served edible flowers before at other restaurants in the Southern California area. Of course, our relatives found this very difficult to believe. Coming from Cleveland, they had never heard of such a thing. As the saying goes, "Only in California." Needless to say, that was a very memorable Sunday brunch for all of us.

CHAPTER SEVENTEEN

There are so many complicated personal and social issues that I was facing during that time as well as today. People simply do not understand the complexity of my problem with the kidneys, and the reason for that is because, out of my own self-consciousness, I do not make an issue of it. But I have to admit that it was very hurtful to me the way some people would just simply gloss over the fact of what is actually wrong with me, almost as though nothing at all were wrong. Perhaps if I didn't appear to look as healthy as I do, they wouldn't act the way they act and it would not appear that way to me.

There have been occasions when we'd be discussing matters involving the illness or a disability of certain members of our family, and either my husband or myself would begin speaking about my experience with lung and liver cancer and something related thereto. Neither one of us would have brought the subject up had we all not been talking about another person's problem. We simply did not want to burden someone by talking about my illness. I especially would not want to ever draw attention to myself in that respect unless somebody asked me a question about it. If that were the case, I would be more than happy to answer any questions or talk about any part of my illness the person making the query wanted to know. The truth is that ninety-nine times out of one hundred the people we were trying to discuss this matter with would listen politely for sixty seconds, if that long, and then immediately change the subject and begin talking about a problem somebody else was experiencing, or a problem that they themselves were experiencing, completely ignoring any words that may have just been spoken by me or my husband. I don't know what it is. For some reason people do not want to hear what you have to say. Maybe they're simply wrapped up in their own problems, their own lives. Nevertheless that's how it happened, and on many more than one occasion. It was rude of them not to let either my husband or me finish what it was we had begun to talk about. The point I'm making is that, hands down, they simply did not want to hear it, and still to this day do not want to hear it. This same reaction has been experienced by every one of the members of my cancer support group, so it is evidently a common occurrence among cancer survivors.

CHAPTER EIGHTEEN

I don't know what I expected when we first arrived back east, but it was obviously something that was not forthcoming. After I'd suffered silently so many times from thinking that friends or relatives were not the least bit concerned about my newly discovered renal condition, I came to the realization that it was because they did not understand it. But I believe they began to understand a little bit more as time went by. Of course, my husband and I are intimately familiar with my problem, and we've adjusted our lives to accommodate it.

Because of people's initial lack of understanding and my not wanting to draw attention to the matter, as previously mentioned, I devised making up my meals ahead of time and taking them along with me whenever we're invited to someone's house for dinner.

In spite of the time that Dr. Sandburg informed me when I first began to see him in California that we had to get my potassium under control or it was possible that one day without warning my heart would just simply stop beating, even then I'm not quite certain that I grasped the seriousness of my chronic kidney failure. However, the seriousness of my condition became very real to me after we moved back east and I applied for Social Security disability, gave the authorities all of the detailed information they requested from me in order to file the claim, and without even challenging me whatsoever they approved my claim. My first check arrived less than a month after my meeting with the local Social Security office. Filing a claim for disability is something I should have done two years earlier before leaving California, but at that time I was not aware that I qualified for disability. Not until we moved back east and a dear friend of ours who also had undergone cancer treatment told me that she was receiving disability payments every month, and she suggested that I attempt to file a claim.

CHAPTER NINETEEN

I believe the straw that broke the camel's back, so to speak, and that which inspired me to begin to prepare my meals ahead of time happened during a weekend that we spent with relatives who live out of town. A couple of weeks prior to our leaving home our niece had asked me via e-mail what I could eat and what I could not eat so that she and her mother would be aware of what foods to shop for. I wrote back via e-mail and sent her a very detailed list of what foods I could eat and what foods were forbidden. I thought how considerate it was of her to ask, and because she did so I was certain that I wouldn't have to worry about a thing once we arrived at their home, nor would I have to undergo further indignation on the subject.

Soon after our arrival on the designated Saturday we were ushered out to the supermarket. I was thinking that Joe and I were to go along to keep my sister-in-law and our niece company; and we were looking forward to touring the beautiful, large, full-service supermarket, something we do not see enough of where we presently live. Not so.

My sister-in-law came up to me and wanted me to walk along beside her in the produce department, telling her what fruits and vegetables I could have, what I could not have and so on and so forth. I was somewhat surprised at her request because of the e-mail transactions that had taken place between our niece and myself prior to our visit.

In order to answer our niece's query, I had done a good deal of research to put together a comprehensive list of good foods versus the bad ones. Please understand that I had been experiencing somewhat similar instances here at home at the aforementioned family get-togethers whereby I became understandably frustrated because I could not find something that I was able to eat on those occasions. Hindsight is always preferable to foresight. It would have been better had I eaten before leaving home, which is what I am prone to do now if I am not taking one of my prepared dinners along with me.

Bear in mind that when you've been through all that I had been through, one's emotions are extremely unstable and always on the surface just waiting to be exposed for the slightest reason, let alone an incident such as this one, which in my estimation was more than slight. Believe me, it does not take a lot to trigger those emotions.

Whenever Joe and I have guests over for dinner, it was and still is always our intention to make them feel as comfortable as possible and to accommodate them in every way that we can so that they do not want for anything once they have arrived at our home. By way of example, if they have a special salad dressing that they enjoy more than others, we always make sure we have it for them, or if somebody happens to be a vegan, we will prepare a vegetarian dish for them, even if our main course for the rest of the guests is porterhouse steak. Before retiring from our jobs, although we both worked long hours during the week and oftentimes on the weekends, especially in my case, I would always take care of whatever needed to be done before our guests' arrival. My husband and I are not in a special category by any means. Everybody in our circle of friends treated us in a like manner. Perhaps I unjustifiably may have hoped for similar treatment on the occasion of our weekend visit.

At the supermarket this particular Saturday I became inwardly and somewhat outwardly annoyed because I thought we had taken care of exchanging all of that information prior to our visit. Rehashing what had already transpired via e-mail and having to talk about what I can and cannot eat again was very uncomfortable for me. Ultimately it served to remind me of my disability, the fact that I am not normal even though I appear to look normal, and that I can no longer enjoy all the wonderful foods that everyone else can enjoy and that I used to take for granted. I was still coming to grips with my disability at the time all of this transpired.

So when my sister-in-law asked me that question, my emotions rose immediately to the surface, I became extremely disappointed, I got a lump in my throat, and I literally could not bring myself to answer her. I went over to where my husband was and I told him that I'd be outside of the store, that I needed some fresh air, which was the truth.

When Joe came outside I told him what had transpired between his sister and me, and he knew at once that I was very upset; so he began to comfort me, assuring me that she had meant no harm. I told him that I was well aware that she had meant no harm, but that really was not the point, and I reminded him of the e-mails that had taken place between our niece and me two weeks prior to this. After a few minutes I went back inside and spent the rest of the time scanning the aisles with our niece, trying to enjoy the privilege of being in a beautiful full-service supermarket once again such as the ones we had left behind in California.

The weekend turned out to be a beautiful one after all in spite of our little exchange or lack thereof in the produce department.

As stated earlier, I have since learned to prepare my own meals ahead of time and take them with me and/or eat before I go to an event or go out of town for a visit, thus avoiding discomfort on anybody's part.

I believe, after many pitfalls and numerous unforeseen difficulties, I have adjusted very well to my new lifestyle of having to follow the renal diet to the letter. It is a small price to pay.

CHAPTER TWENTY

The oncologist whom I began seeing when we moved back east is Dr. James Roberts. He is taking excellent care of me, and I feel very privileged to have found him. When I first began my visits with Dr. Roberts, he saw me every six months at which time he prescribed blood work, of course, a chest X-ray, and then once a year I would have a CT scan of the lung and abdominal area.

During my visit on January 6 of this year, 2006, Dr. Roberts said he was pleased to inform me that I was doing well enough to return for a yearly visit instead of every six months as I had been doing since 2001. Of course, I was thrilled to hear this, and am looking forward to my follow-up visit in January of next year.

CHAPTER TWENTY-ONE

What is gout? The Arthritis Foundation describes it as a disease that causes sudden, severe episodes of pain, tenderness, redness, warmth and swelling (inflammation) in some joints. It usually affects one joint at a time, often the large joint of the big toe. It can also affect other joints, such as the knee, ankle, foot, hand, wrist and elbow. According to the Mayo Clinic, more than two million people are afflicted with this form of arthritis and ninety-five per cent of those are men between forty and fifty. I happened to be misfortunate enough to fall into that five per cent category.

Gout generally occurs in three phases:

1. Sudden joint pain and swelling that usually goes away after five to ten days.

2. A period of no symptoms at all, followed by other acute episodes.

3. After a number of years, if left untreated, persistent swelling, stiffness and mild to moderate pain in one or more joints can occur after numerous acute episodes.

As happened with me each time I experienced an attack, gout episodes usually develop very quickly. The first one often occurs at night. You may go to bed feeling perfectly fine, and wake up with a horrible pain in your joint. This, too, happened to me on more than one occasion.

I woke up one morning in October of 2004 with a swollen, aching right foot which was also a reddish purpleish color at the large joint of the big toe, and the skin was shiny. All of these symptoms I learned later were symptoms of a gout attack. At the time, however, I couldn't imagine what I'd done in order for my foot to be so awfully swollen and sore. The pain was unbelievable, got progressively worse, until it was almost unbearable, and I could not tolerate putting any weight on it.

As the first day that I experienced a gout attack progressed, my foot swelled even more, the swelling extending up into the ankle, and the pain became more and more intolerable with each passing minute. My husband asked me if I wanted to go to the emergency room to have them look at my foot. I said no, that I would see what developed. I remember thinking that maybe, just maybe, the pain would lessen and it would eventually go away for good. Of course, that was wishful thinking on my part, to say the least.

Why do we humans abuse ourselves like that? We always seem to think some miracle will happen and the pain will somehow disappear as quickly as it came. As in this case, that usually never happens, then we end up suffering until we can be seen by a physician and then given the proper treatment. Of course, this first episode of a gout attack occurred on a weekend when doctors are not readily available, with the exception, of course, of the emergency room. As I said, I was hoping above all hope that it would get better on its own. Very often when we need our doctors the most, whatever caused us to be in that position of need has occurred on a weekend. What else would you expect; right? That's Murphy's Law.

I endured the discomfort until Monday when I placed a call to our orthopedist. The reason I called our orthopedist instead of our general practitioner is because I honestly thought that this was a bone-related problem and that somehow I had injured a bone or bones in my foot. I had done something similar to myself in Huntington Beach by stepping on a sharp pebble one summer before we left California, and it took a very long time for my foot to heal before I could put my full weight on it again, so it wasn't entirely out of the question that I could have done something similar to that incident.

Dr. Lawrence had treated me for a fractured clavicle when we first arrived in our new home, and I was extremely pleased with his care. He also had done hip-replacement surgery on my husband the first January after our arrival here on the East Coast. That surgery was very successful, and Joe was pleased with the results; so my faith in Dr. Lawrence's ability to get to the bottom of the problem and get the job done had been established.

I placed a call to Dr. Lawrence's office, and I remember that I was able to get in to see him relatively soon because I explained my dilemma to Lynette, his office manager, with emphasis on the pain I'd been experiencing since awakening that prior Saturday morning. By the time I talked to Lynette the anguish and emotional distress was causing me to be on the verge of tears constantly, first of all due to the intensity of the pain itself, and secondly because by Monday I had become somewhat of an emotional wreck because I thought surely by then that my foot would have been better. So all I needed to do was start explaining to her what was happening to me, when there came the tears gushing out of my eyes, just like Niagara Falls. I was very grateful that she had me come in right away.

At the time I finally placed the call and spoke with Lynette, my right foot had swollen half again the size that it was to start with. As a rule I have very slim feet, for my large frame anyway, and what I was seeing whenever I looked at my right foot and ankle was something bordering on grotesque. There wasn't any way on this earth that I could fit my foot into a shoe, or even one of my soft, sheepskin slippers for that matter. The foot was simply much too swollen.

When I stepped on that sharp pebble in Huntington Beach and my foot swelled up, the podiatrist I saw gave me an orthopedic shoe to wear. It had a very wide foot bed, and you simply laced the shoestring up and tied it at the top, leaving it as loose as is comfortable for your sore foot. Well, let me tell you, that little orthopedic shoe was to come in very handy during the next sixteen months because I would resort to wearing it every time I had a gout attack in either one of my feet. As I was to find out, it wasn't particular which foot the gout attacked, the right or the left, or which of my knees it attacked.

When I saw Dr. Lawrence that Monday morning he took one look at my red, swollen, shiny foot and ankle, and after a long discussion and a very gingerly examination because I could not bear him touching my foot and trying to move it around, he said that it looked like gout. He had me go downstairs to the lab for blood work, which confirmed that the content of my uric acid level was exceptionally high and that it definitely was gout. The reason for the high uric acid content was, of course, my chronic kidney failure.

Normal kidneys would have no trouble processing the uric acid out of the system. According to the Arthritis Foundation, almost all people who have gout have too much uric acid in their blood, a condition called hyperuricemia. The way Dr. Sandburg, my nephrologist in Huntington Beach, explained my condition to me is that I have approximately one-third the use of my kidneys that a normal person has, or that I used to have before I received chemotherapy treatment for lung and liver cancer.

Dr. Lawrence said there were a number of drugs he could recommend for the gout attack I was having, some of which would take care of the problem within a few days. But, of course, I have chronic kidney failure as a result of chemotherapy, which I reminded Dr. Lawrence of, and there are a number of drugs I cannot take because their contra-indications indicate that they are very harmful to the kidneys. My goal is to protect in every way that is humanly possible the one-third use of my kidneys that I have remaining. You could say that I'm overly protective of these internal organs of mine, and I would agree with you one hundred percent. Thus the reason for the ever diligent regime in following my renal diet because I surely do not want to end up having to undergo dialysis, and I've been told that would be the ultimate result of failing to adhere to my renal diet, that or my heart suddenly stopping because of an overabundance of potassium in my system.

After our discussion about the situation with my kidneys, Dr. Lawrence placed a call to Dr. Martin, my nephrologist in Morgantown, and between the two of them they decided that Prednisone would be the drug of choice that I would take to, hopefully, relieve the gout symptoms. I remember that after a few days of taking the Prednisone the gout symptoms appeared to subside a little, and after a few more days the symptoms disappeared and my right foot and ankle appeared to get back to a normal size again.

Then what happened next was that the foot pain and overall gout symptoms shifted from my right foot and ankle to my left foot and ankle. This occurred a day or two after the first gout attack subsided.

While having a gout attack it's next to impossible to do any standing or walking without an aid, and I quickly learned that even having the walker did not allow me to put any weight on the affected foot.

I was fortunate that my husband had been prescribed a walker after his hip-replacement surgery; and when he asked me if I wanted to use the walker, I quickly accepted. I also purchased a cane because once I began to motivate a little bit during these gout attacks and go out with my husband, say, to church or to a relative's house for a visit, or to a Women's Club meeting at the church where I happened to be secretary, or to my Cancer Support Group meetings once a month, it was absolutely essential that I had assistance when walking. Actually, it could be described more as hobbling along than walking. Once the swelling began to subside somewhat during these gout attacks, if the affected foot happened to be my right one, I would then be able to drive myself to and fro.

It was difficult to walk or stand even with my husband's walker because I would have to elevate the affected foot and literally hop on the good foot, being careful not to fall, while holding tightly onto the walker. During the night I'd have to get up one to maybe three times to go to the bathroom to urinate; and getting from the bed to the bathroom was not far, by any means, but having to hobble on one foot, even with the aid of the walker, to go to the bathroom was cumbersome, to say the least, and extremely painful. During these times I would trade places with Joe because his side of the bed is a good deal closer to the master bathroom; this meant I would only have to maneuver a few feet when I had to get up in the middle of the night to answer Nature's call.

The anguish that a person has to endure when a gout attack occurs is indescribable. Actually, a friend of ours who also experiences gout attacks said that when an attack occurs, in his opinion, even a cool breeze blowing softly against the foot will cause excruciating pain. We can laugh about it when we're free of any attacks, but what he said makes every bit of sense in the world to a person afflicted with this disease. It's for certain you cannot tolerate a sheet or, heaven forbid, a blanket resting on your foot. Putting your foot into a shoe is impossible, even a soft, fuzzy slipper. First of all, the foot becomes so very swollen that it would never fit through the opening, and secondly, the pain, if you could squeeze the foot into the shoe or slipper, would be so intensely unpleasant that you could not bear it.

During these gout attacks for the most part I was unable to attend church on Sundays, nor could I do the mundane chores that are necessary in every household such as grocery shopping, preparing meals, doing the laundry, ironing, and keeping the house in order. I had been a faithful bi-weekly attendee at the local YMCA for three years standing, and I was unable to go there from September of 2004 until June of 2006. I enjoyed the water aerobics class and going into the gym afterwards to do one circuit on the Nautilus machines, followed by a two-mile walk on the treadmill. However, I simply could not stand nor motivate without the affected foot, knee, or both at one time throbbing and driving me wild with pain. When the gout attacked my right foot, in the early stages of the attack I could not drive, therefore, I was housebound and not liking it one bit. I've always enjoyed driving to town either to visit a friend, going to the mall, or being able to do the grocery shopping if it happened to be time to do so.

Being immobile and keeping my foot elevated on a pillow and iced down was what Dr. Lawrence suggested I do. It really didn't give me much relief. Nothing did. Even when I slept, any movement whatsoever that I made involving the affected area would be very painful and would wake me out of a sound sleep. The only relief I did experience was when the gout attack subsided. What a glorious time that was.

From the period October 23, 2004, to February 11, 2006, I had twenty gout attacks, some of them back-to-back, and some which lasted two weeks or longer. One attack in particular lasted three whole weeks. There were times that I became so distraught that I thought I would lose my mind.

My husband took over the kitchen duties along with the other household duties that I've mentioned here. He is a very devoted, kind man, is sympathetic, warm, attentive, caring, and loving. He did everything in his power to make me comfortable. He's a wonderful cook, also. I've been blessed in many ways, and having a mate like him is right up there in the top ten.

Joe had surgery to repair his rotator cuff the morning of October 10, 2005. I woke up that morning with unbearable pain in my right knee. It was extremely swollen and tender to the touch. I could not bend it, nor move it without wanting to scream aloud. Joe's sister Celine and a good friend of ours, Alan Prescott, were kind enough to sit with me in the waiting room while Joe underwent surgery which was performed by Dr.

Lawrence. Because of the pain I was experiencing in my right knee, I had taken my cane along with me to the hospital, but it did not alleviate the difficulty I experienced trying to sit down or to rise from a seated position. The difficulty stemmed from not being able to bend my knee because of the pain, not to mention the fact that it was swollen and frozen stiff.

After Joe's surgery Dr. Lawrence came to the waiting room and informed me that my husband was in recovery, he was doing well, he would be in his room in about thirty minutes, the surgery was a success, and, by the way, what was the matter with my knee. He asked me if the gout had returned. I told him that I certainly hoped it was not gout this time. He said to come and see him in the afternoon; and I said I would be there, and that I'd already called Lynette, his secretary, to set up an appointment. If it were not for Alan assisting me across the hospital grounds to the building where Dr. Lawrence was located, I don't think I would have made it. Yes, I had the aid of my cane, but holding on to Alan's arm and his catching me and stopping me from falling when my knee gave out and I almost lost my balance was truly a lifesaver.

When I saw Dr. Lawrence later that afternoon, after talking with me and a thorough examination he said he thought it was the gout again. He injected my swollen knee with a needle and he drained the liquid off my knee which had developed there, sent it to the lab for analysis, and then he called me later that day to inform me that, indeed, it was gout. He then prescribed some medication for me to take once again, hopefully, to ease the inflammation.

Having gout in the knee was a totally new experience, like none other. When you think about how many times a day you bend your knees, it's unconscionable to imagine having gout in your knee and not being able to bend it without experiencing immeasurable pain with every insignificant movement. We move our knees without even thinking about what we're doing: sitting; standing; getting in bed; getting out of bed; getting comfortable while in bed; crossing your legs, stepping over the little stoop to get into and out of the shower; getting in and out of the car; going to the bathroom; getting to the bathroom in order to go to the bathroom. With the exception of that period of time during the middle of the night, I found that using our guest bathroom was by far the most convenient for me because it's quite a bit larger than our small closet toilet in our master bathroom where it was not near as roomy. In the guest bathroom I found that I could stretch my leg out and not have to worry about its possible bending at any given time, plus I could grab hold of the sink on my right and the rim of the bathtub on my left to assist me in getting up and down. The whole scenario was dreadful.

I was having so many gout attacks, one right after another, because, obviously the medicines that I was prescribed were not taking care of the problem. One medicine in particular, Colchicine, made me so sick with stomach aches and diarrhea that I was happy to finally be rid of it. I remember being at a Women's Club meeting at our church where I was busily taking notes because that was my job as secretary, a throwback to my court reporting days, no doubt, when suddenly the "urge" came over me, and I had to get up and proceed to the ladies room which was a good distance down the hallway, hobbling along slowly with the aid of my cane because the pain I was enduring wouldn't allow me to move as quickly as I would have liked. I have not taken that particular drug since then.

Finally in February of 2006 I was prescribed 150 milligrams of Allopurinal, which I'm to take daily for the rest of my life, and which, in my humble opinion, is a wonder drug. As described by the Arthritis Foundation, "Allopurinol reduces the amount of uric acid in your blood and urine by slowing the rate at which the body makes uric acid. It is the best medicine for people who have kidney problems." It is responsible for keeping the gout at bay, and it does a remarkable job of doing just that. I have been able to experience peace of mind, body and soul at last, and since

I've started taking this wonder drug, I have been gout-free. Why I was not prescribed Allopurinal before then is anybody's guess.

Having to follow the renal diet to the letter was bad enough, but in addition to that I am obligated to follow a diet geared towards keeping me gout-free. However, it's not the end of the world, and I shall persevere. Some of the foods I am to avoid or to ingest in moderation since I've begun to have gout attacks are red meat, bacon, asparagus, kidney beans, lima beans, mushrooms, spinach, cauliflower, anchovies, legumes, and all shellfish. These foods tend to increase blood uric acid levels.

Beer is the alcoholic beverage which is the worst offender to precipitate a gout attack. Wine is the least. Foods which may be beneficial to gout patients are dark berries because they may contain chemicals that lower uric acid and also reduce inflammation, tofu, which I cannot eat because of my chronic kidney failure, and pineapple. There are many foods which are allowed on the gout diet which are not allowed on the renal diet, so I am very careful to watch what I eat.

All in all, life is good. I'm happy to be alive and to be able to enjoy all the blessings that God has bestowed upon me, not to mention being able to take pleasure in nature's beautiful creatures that are abundant here in the hills of West Virginia, such as the energetic and graceful purple martins which we've built a birdhouse for and who reside in our back yard during the spring and summer months. They're so lovely to watch as they fly to and fro, searching for the bugs which give them sustenance. Then there are the yellow finches, the blue birds, the woodpeckers, the blue jays, the orioles, the ducks, the families of geese and their goslings, even the sparrows, all of which we provide food for. And the hummingbirds. We cannot forget the beautiful little hummingbirds who fight as though there's no tomorrow over the two feeders we keep filled on our front porch. Joe and I spend hours together watching these miracles of nature.

Speaking of miracles, that is the way I look upon myself now, having survived small-cell metastatic carcinoma of the lung and liver, a cancer which has only a ten percent survival rate.

Finding myself in that elite group of ten per cent, I believe I truly am the result of a miracle.

Printed in the United States
145716LV00004B/75/A